Operative Obstetrics

Second Edition

Major changes in obstetric practice have occurred in the ten years since the publication of the first edition of *Operative Obstetrics*. Prospective clinical studies have improved clinical practice, and better techniques for antenatal fetal evaluation have been introduced. Yet, there are also less desirable trends. There has been a relentless increase in the rate of cesarean delivery, and persisting medicolegal and societal pressures continue to demand faultless performance. Our recognition of recent improvements in clinical practice and acknowledgement of the continuing challenges and limitations inherent in modern clinical management have prompted a new edition. This updated edition includes chapters on the important subjects of cesarean delivery, common surgical complications, ectopic pregnancy, birth injury, and instrumental delivery, among other topics. It features a new discussion of surgical procedures performed by non-physicians and a review of fetal surgery. The text also considers complicated and controversial subjects such as cervical insufficiency, pregnancy termination, and shoulder dystocia. In recognition of the realities of current practice, each of the four sections of the book has a chapter with an in-depth analysis of the legal issues underlying practice. An expanded appendix reviews general legal concepts pertinent to the practice of obstetrics.

John P. O'Grady is professor of obstetrics and gynecology at the Tufts University School of Medicine, Boston, Massachusetts. He is medical director of the Family Life Center for Maternity and heads the Perinatal Service at Mercy Medical Center in Springfield, Massachusetts. He graduated from Yale University School of Medicine and has published a number of books in the field of obstetrics.

Martin L. Gimovsky is clinical professor of obstetrics and gynecology at the Mount Sinai School of Medicine in New York. A graduate of the New York University School of Medicine, he is Residency Program Director for the Department of Obstetrics and Gynecology at Newark Beth Israel Medical Center in Newark, New Jersey.